ANNA

150 TIPS FOR EVERYDAY LIVING WITH ME/CFS

The information and opinions presented in this book are believed to be accurate and sound, based on the best judgement available to the author and publisher, but readers assume the risk of any loss, injuries or damage caused by following the advice contained here. Readers should consult a physician in relation to any matters pertaining to their health. All information is believed to be accurate at the time of writing.

Published July 2013

Copyright © 2013 Anna Cayder
All rights reserved

Cover Photo: gerisima/iStockphoto

No part of this book may be reproduced in any format except for the use of brief quotations in a book review. The author has worked long and hard to produce this book. Please respect that and do not breach copyright.

*To all my fellow patients
and the family, friends,
doctors and researchers
who support us.*

CONTENTS

1. Introduction 1

2. General Strategies 5

3. Personal Care 13
   Care of your teeth 13
   Bathing 15
   Haircare 17
   Grooming 22

4. In the kitchen 23
   Cooking 23
   Arranging and using the kitchen 28
   Kitchen equipment 30
   Washing up 32

5. Housework 35
   General cleaning 35
   Floors 37
   Laundry 40
   Ironing 42
   Changing bedlinen 44

6. Other activities in the home 47
Shopping from home..47
Walking and carrying..51
Visitors..54
Using the phone 55
Reading..56
Household Emergencies 59

7. Out and About...61
Shopping outside the home..............................61
Appointments 63
Travel and mobility 66
Resting outdoors 69

8. Three last general strategies....................................71

9. Reasons to be cheerful..73

1. INTRODUCTION

Last year, after decades of experience of using all sorts of dodges to cope with the limitations caused by having ME, I thought I'd knock off a quick list of 50 or so helpful tips for saving your energy, and publish it. After all, I've had ME for most of my adult life, slowly improving from being bedbound to being able to cope with independent though mostly housebound living. I assumed I already knew everything there was to know about how to survive with the least possible effort.

But I thought I'd better check, so I started consulting other sources: other ME patients, books on housework avoidance, medical charity websites, internet forums for people with all sorts of debilitating illnesses, you name it. As I discovered one 'why didn't I think of that 20 years ago' idea after another, my working title changed from '50 Tips for Everyday Living with ME/CFS' to '100 Tips', then '150 Tips'. It should now really be '188 Tips' but I thought that would just look weird. I've found so much new and useful information despite my quarter-century experience of ME that I've had to print off the list of tips and use a magic marker to highlight the new things I want to try myself.

I hope you'll discover some new tips too, but without quite so much forehead-slapping.

Who this book is for

The tips in this volume are aimed at people who need to save their energy, because with ME even trivial effort can cause severe fatigue and worsen other symptoms. Different tips apply to different levels of ability: there are ideas to help everyone from the bedbound to those able to sporadically do light housework. Because your energy can vary even from hour to hour you may find some tips useful at one time but not another, whatever your usual level of function.

If you are so ill that you require assisted living, I highly recommend in addition a book by the late Emily Collingridge, *Severe ME/CFS: A Guide to Living*, published by the Association of Young People with ME (AYME) and available from them.

Most suggestions in this book cost nothing while a few are beyond the means of many of us but I've listed them just in case. Almost all of the tips apply wherever you live but the specifics in some cases relate only to the UK.

But whatever your limitations, your means or your location, I hope there'll be plenty of new ideas in here for you!

No web links!

Web links for useful goods and services go out of date quickly so I haven't provided any. Instead, I've suggested web search terms for certain things because they'll never go out of date and they're more useful for an international audience.

Who's paying me?

In my research I've come across a lot of handy products and so I've mentioned them. I'm not getting paid by anybody to promote their stuff and I only vouch personally for what I've actually tried.

How to use this book

Slowly! And, if you've got the paperback version, use a magic marker. Go on, wreck it, it was cheap! It has no resale value! It's meant to be used. And if you have it on an e-reader, use the highlighter function. You'll have forgotten which tips you liked by the time you get to the end.

2. GENERAL STRATEGIES

Before we get down to specific tips, there are some general strategies that apply to all of them.

Accept that you need to adapt, just for now
For the first few years of being ill, I was confined to bed for over 23 hours a day but I resisted lying down completely flat because that would have meant that I was very badly ill. I avoided making a lot of adaptations that would have helped me — hiring some help, getting a shower-seat, cutting my hair shorter so I could manage it — for the same reason. Denial! Great stuff.

I now realise that my reluctance to face the severity of my illness was based on my fear that it was permanent, so the sooner I faced it, the longer I'd have to live with knowing that I was severely disabled and always would be.

After years of being ill without improvement this may be natural but it's not logical. First, the more adaptations you make, the more rest you can get, and the better your chances of recovery. Once I started lying down in bed, I started to improve. Second, after decades of ME being neglected, the research cavalry are finally galloping over the horizon and proper medical help (wow!) may soon be on its way. I'll be saying more about the research in a later chapter.

So, if you adapt to your situation, it doesn't mean it's forever. Because it isn't.

Lower your standards!

As a natural slob, I'm delighted to have a legitimate reason to jettison even the meagre standards of housekeeping that I could be bothered with even before I got sick. You may be different, and if so, it's worth questioning what you do.

Do you iron things? Any things? Do you really care that they're ironed? Does anybody in your house care? If someone in your house cares, shouldn't they be the one doing that ironing? Do you think your visitors notice that there's stuff in your house that you haven't ironed? Do you think they think badly of you for it? Would you think badly of someone who didn't iron things because they were ill?

I haven't ironed anything since 2003 and no-one has ironed anything for me. I couldn't be happier with my lack of pointlessly-ironed stuff. Low standards? Certainly: no standards at all, in fact. Do I care? Clearly not. Does anyone else? If they do, they've never said so. If they did, I'd think they had strange priorities for their very ill friend.

We all have to do our own head-work on this one. Think about what you're doing. Are you vacuum-cleaning every week? Why? Are you drying dishes with a cloth instead of letting them dry naturally? Why? Is it really worth it to you? Are you keeping standards that are more to do with appearances than with keeping your home a healthy place to be?

If you're not sure about letting some of this stuff go, give it a trial period of a week, a month, whatever you like. At the end of that, decide which standards really matter to you and which don't. Come on in, the squalor's lovely!

Get someone else to do it

I'm huge fan of getting someone else to do the housework and cooking. If you live with a family member, that's an obvious source of help. Otherwise, it's a case of getting someone in.

Depending on how much help you need, what your finances are like and where you live, you may be able to get help from your local council. If you can afford it, you can directly hire a cleaner or a home help. Prices vary as to location but whereas cleaners just, well, clean, home helps do a range of work including cleaning and food preparation, as well as help with personal care if that's what you want. As a result, they cost more than cleaners. However, it's up to you how many hours they work: I hire a home help for the minimum hour a week through an agency in a big city and that costs me less than £20. That hour is enough to make sure that on a two-week cycle, my small flat gets its hoovering and dusting done, the kitchen and bathroom get cleaned and the bedding gets changed, plus there's a bit of food preparation to set me up for each week ahead.

For me, it's well worth it; and if you're ill enough to need that help and live in the UK, you are probably ill enough to get Disability Living Allowance (now being replaced by the Personal Independence Payment), which will cover at least some of the cost.

It might seem a bit grim to have to hire a home help, especially if you're relatively young. I didn't realise the range of work that home helps did until my 83-year-old father needed one and then I realised that I could use similar help myself! But I'm finding it's a lot nicer to have a clean house and enough spare energy to go out for coffee, than not to have a home help.

Again, it's not forever, and you can have a go for a trial period and cancel the contract if you don't like it.

Little and not all that often

With ME, it's very important to pace your daily activities. Not only does that mean spreading activities out across the day — or across several days — it may mean breaking what would normally be a single activity into bits, with breaks between.

For example, in normal health you'd unload the dishwasher in one go. With ME, you might be better off unloading it a bit at a time, with rests in between. Previously, you might have had a shower and washed your hair at the same time. Now, you might wash your hair in the morning but shower in the evening. You might once have done all the washing up in one go: now, maybe it's the cutlery first and the other stuff later. You could try setting a timer for five minutes, say, of activity and then stop and come back to the task later.

You might also benefit from just doing some activities less often. When in the past you might have cleaned the bathroom sink once a week, now you might do it once a fortnight, or less.

Little, and less often.

Time harder activities for when you have more energy
You may have noticed that you're better at certain times of the day. If so, save activities that you struggle with for these times.

Sit down and put your feet up
Some studies indicate that as many as 97% of people with ME have problems with regulating their heart rate and/or blood pressure when sitting or standing. They don't necessarily feel dizzy or faint, but they become rapidly fatigued and eventually need to lie down; they often find it easier to keep walking than to stand still, though both exhaust them. This condition is called orthostatic intolerance, and you may have heard it mentioned in one of its specific forms; POTS (postural orthostatic tachycardia syndrome) or NMH (neurally mediated hypotension).

If you find standing particularly tiring, this could be why, and you may find it helps to sit, or sit with your feet up, as much as possible while doing tasks. For example, try sitting at a table to chop vegetables rather than standing at the kitchen counter, and close the loo seat and sit there while you're cleaning your teeth instead of standing at the basin.

Keep your arms below your heart
For many people with orthostatic intolerance, raising or keeping their arms above heart-level can make them feel worse very quickly. Let someone else hang those curtains!

Think the unthinkable: energy vs cost
If you don't have much money, or just have frugal habits, it can be hard to adjust your ideas to spending money on

things that would seem like luxuries in good health but that can be necessities when you're ill.

My own blind spot until recently was taxis. When I was well, I'd walk miles rather than cough up for a taxi but now, their occasional and judicious use make a trip to the town centre possible when it would have been exhausting by bus. Another thing for me was the idea of hiring help at home. I have friends who have cleaners and it always seemed like the sort of thing the aristocracy would do. Not any more!

So, reconsider a few things: are they still luxuries or do your circumstances now justify them?

Prioritise

The only two fillings I've ever needed in my life were the year I was too ill to clean my teeth every day. In contrast, your ankles won't drop off if you don't wash them for a year. Prioritise! Put health and survival over appearance every time.

Seek out product reviews

I mention a number of products in this book that you might find helpful but I can only vouch for the ones I've tried, and even then, only for the particular item that I bought and not the other 100,000 that the factory turned out. If you're going to buy some potentially useful item, particularly something expensive, check out reviews and pay particular attention to critical ones. I look at reviews on Amazon and although I'm in the UK, often look at the reviews on the US Amazon site because America has a much bigger population and hence more people reviewing products. Be sceptical — these are the days of industry-sponsored sock-puppets leaving positive reviews for their companies' own products — and consider looking at review sources that are independent, such as *Which?* magazine.

So, preamble over. Now onto individual tasks!

3. PERSONAL CARE

Care of your teeth

Avoid repeated exposure to sugary things
It's not how much sugar you eat, it's how many sugar attacks a day your teeth get that determine how rapidly they decay. Plaque bacteria produce acid from sugar for about 20 minutes after you've had some; obviously if you eat sugar more often, that's more time that your tooth enamel is being nibbled by acid. Avoid repeatedly eating or drinking sugary things to help prevent problems and save you an exhausting trip to the dentist.

Use an electric toothbrush
An electric toothbrush saves wearing your arm out and, unless you're some sort of ninja expert in manual brushing, will clean your teeth better. Highly recommended.

Use interdental brushes
If you struggle with using dental floss, have a go with Tepe interdental brushes. Each one is a small brush like a tiny pipecleaner that you shove between your teeth instead of

flossing. You buy them in packets of half a dozen or more, and dispose of them after a few uses.

Change your teeth-cleaning posture

Standing to clean your teeth may tire you, particularly because to clean your teeth you've got to keep your arms higher than your heart so you may be especially far into orthostatic intolerance territory.

Try sitting while cleaning your teeth or, if necessary, get your feet up. If you can't do that in the bathroom, bring the brush, toothpaste, an empty container to spit in and a glass of water and do your teeth-cleaning in a less tiring position, such as sitting in an armchair with your feet up or while sitting up in bed.

Get some help

It never occurred to me to ask for help when I was too ill to clean my teeth in the bathroom. If you have someone available, get them to put some toothpaste onto a dry brush and bring it and the other paraphernalia to you.

Use bare-minimum teeth-cleaning in emergencies

Brush your teeth morning and night every day if you can, but on those occasions when you can't, at least floss — which you can do while reclining, most easily with a Tepe interdental brush — and dry-brush your teeth without toothpaste.

Get the community dentist to visit

If you live in the UK and you're completely housebound you can ask your GP to refer you to the community dental service who will be able to check your teeth at home.

Bathing

Reconsider your bathing routine
If it has been your lifelong habit to bathe in the morning, it can be strangely unthinkable to do it at another time of day. However, if you find this task difficult, it might be best to change your routine so that you're doing it when you tend to have more energy. I shower in the evening these days because I feel better then and I don't have to face it in the morning when I'm not so good.

Try cooler water
Some people with ME find hot showers or baths exhausting. Try them cooler.

Use a shower seat
I wish I'd known about these years ago. You can get a shower bench, which sits across the sides of the bath and is secured by rubber grippers; or a shower stool or seat with non-slip feet that sits on the floor of the bath or shower; or a fold-down seat that is attached to your shower wall. They're not all that expensive considering how useful they are: about £25 upwards at the time of writing. You don't have to go to a specialist shop to get one, either. Just type 'shower seat' into Amazon or Ebay and you're laughing.

To wash your hair, sit on the seat and lower your head rather than raising your arms. It's likely to be much less tiring.

Use the shower handset
You might find it easier to detach the handset from its holder and bring it to you while you're sitting on a shower seat, rather than standing under the showerhead.

Have a sponge bath
If a shower is too much to cope with on any particular day, just a wash using a flannel or a sponge is an option. You may be too tired to wash all over, in which case, you could concentrate on the bits that are important. You know the bits I mean…

Use wet-wipes, alcohol wipes or no-rinse cleanser
If even a sponge bath is off the menu, then wet-wipes or scent-free alcohol wipes are an option. They kill germs that cause odour so help keep you fresh. There is also a product that comes in a bottle, called No Rinse Body Bath, developed for astronauts, that's alcohol-free and so doesn't dry out your skin and doesn't — surprise! — need rinsing.

Sit down to towel-dry
Dry yourself off sitting on a shower bench or on the closed loo seat. It's just easier.

Use a towelling robe to get dry
Sitting in a terrycloth robe to dry takes much less effort than scrubbing away with a towel.

Use a microfibre bath towel
Questionable, this one. On the one hand, microfibre towelling is extremely lightweight and absorbent so should be less work than using a cotton towel. On the other hand,

microfibre towelling gives some people the willies, and I'm one of them. Online, some people say they're great, and swear by them for the gym and camping; others say they feel kind of creepy, as though you're trying to dry yourself with velvet.

So, you're on your own with this one. If you do decide to try one, apparently you have to wash them a few times to really get them going. Bear in mind that you shouldn't wash them with other things because the microfibre filaments attract lint, which reduces their effectiveness.

Haircare

Get a haircut that doesn't need styling
Using a blow-dryer can be especially tiring for people with ME who also have orthostatic intolerance because it forces you to have your arms above heart-level. If that's the case for you, try a hairstyle that you can finish by just running a comb, brush, or your hands through it.

Get a shorter haircut
Hair was seen as the crowning glory of the Victorian lady, but if she became seriously ill, her hair got chopped off. Not quite sure what the reasoning was but clearly there's precedent for this idea.

I've found that a shorter haircut has made my hair easier both to wash and to dry. It's a personal choice but it's worth considering.

Get a good haircut
It can be demoralising to be forced by illness to get your hair cut shorter than you're used to, so get some hairstyle magazines and put some effort into finding a fashionable cut that suits your face shape and hair type. Take the photos to a good hairdresser and talk it through before the big chop. My hair looks far better (surprisingly) now that it's short because I put a lot of thought into choosing a good style.

Shave your head
Shaving your head is probably just one for the guys, who knows? But it saves dealing with hair.

Use a mobile hairdresser
...rather than going to a salon. It's a lot cheaper, too.

Use hair clippers
If you have short hair, forget the hairdresser/barber altogether and get some hair clippers. There's some skill to using them, as I can testify, having done a bit of a sheep-shearing job on my dad's head once. Sorry, Dad. I wish I had thought to search for 'hair clippers tutorial' on YouTube: lots of useful videos there.

Basin-wash your hair
Washing both your hair and your body in the shower can be a bit too epic. If so, consider washing your hair in the basin and showering your body at a different time. You can use a showerhead arrangement that fixes to the basin taps; or, as I do, just fill the basin with water, dunk your head in, and change the water for the second rinse.

Use dry shampoo

Dry shampoo is a powder containing cornflour or talc to absorb the oil in your hair. You spray it in and brush or towel-rub it out. It doesn't tend to work as well as ordinary shampoo and can leave a white residue but if you're blonde you might get away with it!

Not ideal, but needs must, sometimes. Some people simply use cornflour or talc rather than a manufactured shampoo.

Use no-rinse shampoo

Nilaqua ('no water', geddit?) make a shampoo called No Rinse that doesn't need to be rinsed out, a companion product to its no-rinse body cleanser. Both were originally developed for the NASA space programme but are now used in a more pedestrian manner by campers, the ill and the elderly. You apply the shampoo until your hair is wet, massage it to a lather and thoroughly towel dry without rinsing. The shampoo releases the dirt and oil from your scalp into the lather and the towel absorbs that lather.

I saw a concern raised online that No Rinse shampoo contained progesterone (a hormone that you wouldn't want to be taking in) so I contacted the company. They told me that production of Nilaqua products has returned to the UK and none of their products contain progesterone; they are also free of parabens and alcohol. Overseas customers buying the Nilaqua brand will get the same UK product.

I haven't used it, but now that I've read about it, I fancy it.

There's also a No Rinse Shampoo Cap that you microwave for a few seconds and put on your hair. You then massage your hair through the cap, throw the cap away and towel your hair.

Leave shampoo in for five minutes before rinsing
…to give it a chance to absorb the oils. I read this tip some months ago and have been testing it. I'm not sure if it makes any difference. Perhaps it might for you.

Use a microfibre hair towel
My earlier comments about creepy microfibre towels notwithstanding, any adaptation that reduces the need for blowdrying or helps you to get your hair dry without using lots of soggy towels is good. At least the fabric won't be touching your skin. Urgh!

Use a lightweight hairdryer
Travel hairdryers are often light and thus less tiring to use but if you'd prefer a conventional one, bung 'lightweight hairdryer' into Amazon's search bar and look at the weight in the product description. Wish I'd thought of that a month ago when I replaced my broken hairdryer.

Use a hands-free hairdryer
Who knew these existed? Not me, until I started researching this book, that's for sure. You can get either a hands-free dryer with a clip that attaches to a wall, or buy a floor-stand or table-top stand in which you can place your present dryer. Amazing.

Some customer reviews suggest that certain models struggle with heavier hairdryers, so read the reviews and if you get one you're not happy with, send it back.

Lean forward to dry your hair

If keeping your arms raised tires you, lean forward to blow-dry your hair so that you don't have to hold the dryer so high.

Train your hair to need less washing

It's possible to train your hair to need washing less frequently. It's my ambition in this book to avoid squalor — well, too much squalor, anyway — but there may be some short-lived dismalness in implementing this suggestion. On the other hand, there's a big potential pay-off in cutting down on a tiring task.

The scalp produces oil in response to being stripped of it, so the more you wash your hair, the more oil your hair will produce. Try leaving your hair without washing a day longer than usual for a few weeks and see if it starts to need it less. Scrubbing your scalp while you're shampooing also encourages the production of oil (I now learn, after decades of scrubbing at my scalp) so avoid that too.

Some people wash their hair just in water, without shampoo, and find that much easier to live with than not washing their hair at all. However, both the no-shampoo and the washing-less-often methods of hair-training don't seem to work for everyone and for those for whom it does work, there's a transition period of some weeks (six weeks being an oft-quoted figure) before your hair gets the message.

There's a huge range of opinion on the net about not using shampoo. For some people it works, and for others it doesn't. Until that happy day when somebody does a proper trial of it on a lot of people, it's a matter of experimenting for yourself.

Grooming

Use less or no make-up
A tip for the girls, or possibly also the guys, I'm not judging: it's tiring to put slap on and take it off again so either do without, or only use the make-up you can't bear to do without.

Don't shave bits that don't need shaving
Legs and underarms, ladies! If you're not waving them about in public, don't bother shaving them. Wear trousers! And long-sleeved stuff!

4. IN THE KITCHEN

Cooking

Eat no-prep food
This is the best kind of cooking! Just take this stuff out of the packet and get stuck in. Nuts, seeds, avocados, cheese, roast meat, marinated tofu, yoghurt, bread, crispbreads, pre-cut carrot sticks, fruit...

Eat ready-meals
If you're careful to select the healthier versions, you can do well with pre-cooked meals that just need re-heating: particularly easy using the microwave.

Eat oven-ready food
When you're used to being unable to cook, it's easy to forget that your oven exists, let alone to remember that everything that goes in it doesn't have to be prepared by you and needn't involve pans and casserole dishes to wash up. Supermarkets do many oven-ready items in foil trays ready for roasting, including vegetable dishes.

Eat low-prep food
Instead of cooking vegetables, eat them raw and dip them in houmous, tzatziki and so on. Some vegetables can be

steamed in the bag: for example, kale from some supermarkets comes in bags that you stab a few enjoyable times and then bung in the microwave. Done!

Prepare one-pot, one-dish meals
Hearty soups and casseroles that contain both meat and vegetables are easier to cook, easier to reheat and need only one bowl so they're easier to wash up.

Use stripped-down recipes
Normal recipes have a lot of ingredients and stages and that's what makes them tiring to prepare. But consider your favourite recipes and what the essential thing about them is that you like. Pasta with mushrooms and thyme? Forget the pasta, have some bread instead and microwave some mushrooms with a bit of thyme.

Websurf for easy recipes
Select a favourite basis for a meal, such as chicken, and search the web using terms such as 'easy chicken recipes' or 'three ingredient chicken recipes'.

Prepare your meal in stages
There's no need to make your whole meal in one go: prepare bits of it at a time. You can either do this in advance, spacing out the tasks, or alternate a bit of preparation with a bit of eating.

Use pre-chopped frozen and fresh vegetables
Whether frozen or fresh, someone has done all the work for you with pre-chopped vegetables so take full advantage.

Prepare ingredients in bulk, not just meals

I find that I can't find some ingredients ready-prepared how I need them and there are some vegetables I find it easier to prepare in bulk in one go while sitting at a table than fiddling about to make one portion at a time. Chopped vegetables keep pretty well in the fridge.

Batch cook

For some recipes that don't involve much preparation of ingredients, making double quantities is no harder than making one portion. For other recipes, it's double the quantity and double the work.

It's worth considering whether any of your cooking falls into the first category and if so, batch cook and refrigerate or freeze extra portions for later.

Check for new food products

Supermarkets are always introducing new products to tempt us, and some of those new things require no or little preparation, so it's worth going online or into the store to see what's new. I recently discovered that Waitrose do pre-peeled onions: just top and tail them and do some minor chopping and you can roast a week's worth. They also offer some (OK, pricey) salmon fillets that are healthily poached in just lemon juice and white wine and ready to eat.

There's all sorts of good stuff waiting to be discovered, and you don't have to stick to one supermarket, either; shop around.

Use a home-delivery meals service

Some companies deliver entire frozen meals to your door. The dishes come as single servings and include vegetable accompaniments so all you do is shove them in the microwave or the oven.

In the UK, Wiltshire Farm Foods and Oakhouse Foods are well-known home-delivery firms and their range doesn't appear to be pitched entirely to the elderly as you might expect. At the posher end, if you fancy salmon mousse with pomegranate seeds and spelt bread with three-leaf salad, there's slimming-meal company Nutrichef, though at around £15 a day, it's not cheap but it is free of artificial additives, wheat and dairy. COOK (I'm not shouting, that's how they write it) is a company that makes dishes from the same ingredients that you would use at home, so again, no weird additives. You can buy their products in one of their 60 shops or order them for home delivery if you're within range. I've tried their stuff and it's great, although the quality is reflected somewhat in the price.

These are just some examples. Google on 'meals home delivery' and see if anything appeals to you within your budget. Remember, you don't have to live off the meals entirely and for most of these services, you just buy as and when you want. If you stock up on their frozen meals you can just use them when you need.

Hire a caterer or personal chef

If you're really pushing the boat out, google for local caterers or personal chefs and ask about having them prepare a shedload of your favourite meals to portion up and put in the freezer. Some people pay a friend, or a hard-up student to do the same job.

Keep stocked up for an emergency

It's wise to prepare for a 'can't get to the shops' or a 'too ill to cook' emergency by stocking up. Make sure you've got ready-meals in the freezer, canned stuff you can just tip into a bowl and microwave, and other things that need no preparation such as oatcakes and crispbread, nuts and nut butters, cheese, tins of sardines, dried fruit and so on.

You can freeze cheese, bread and milk so that you always have an emergency supply. It's handy to have individual portions of things in the freezer so you don't have to deal with defrosting and dividing larger quantities. I have been known to eat frozen peas straight from the bag. Some of these things will be healthy food, some of it will be emergency fuel. You can't be perfect in an emergency, so don't worry about it.

Ask guests to cook for themselves

If you're well enough to have people round for a meal, ask them to bring a course, particularly a main course if you think they'd be happy to. You can provide the easy stuff such as dessert (which you buy rather than make, of course) and wine.

Eat a good enough diet, not a perfect one

When you're ill, it's natural to become focused on your diet as a means to try to get well. Sometimes you might not be able to live up to your highest standards in this regard: come and join me in the breaded fish department.

Arranging and using the kitchen

Avoid using the hob
Having to stand at the hob stirring things, supervising them, hoicking heavy pans around and so on is tiring. Try instead to use the microwave or oven. If you really want to use the hob, cook things that don't need much attention.

Use the microwave rather than the oven
Using the microwave involves less hefting and bending than the oven. Some things don't taste as good done in the microwave as in the oven: it's for you to decide whether the trade-off in terms of effort is worth it.

Avoid food preparation at the counter
Consider what cooking jobs you could do sitting down rather than standing at the counter, such as chopping vegetables. I don't have a kitchen table so I cover my dining table with a plastic tablecloth and use that.

Slide heavy things, don't lift them
Sliding things rather than lifting them is a good technique in general. For example, I use it to unpack bags of heavy groceries; I put the bags on the kitchen counter, pull the sides of the bags down, and slide the contents onto the counter.

Keep often-used things near waist-height
Reaching up and bending low to get things is tiring. You might find it easier to keep frequently used things

permanently out on the counter rather than in cupboards and drawers.

Keep tableware near the table or dishwasher
Tableware moves between your table and your dishwasher (or kitchen sink) so it makes sense to keep it near one of them. Don't move it about more than you have to!

Keep a tray of tea-things on the counter
If people often come by, keep a tray with mugs, cups and so on permanently on the counter.

Keep things together that are used together
Keep pans near the stove, the can opener near the cans, and so on.

Use a towel to catch water when defrosting the freezer
It can be very tiring to get all the melted water out of the bottom of your freezer when you've defrosted it. Before you switch the freezer off, line the bottom with a binbag. It will catch most of the water and you can absorb the rest with a bathroom towel and throw the towel straight into the washing machine.

You can, of course, speed the defrosting process by placing a Pyrex bowl of hot water on a shelf in the freezer, replacing the water as it cools.

Kitchen equipment

Consider helpful gadgets
Ah, gadgets. This one can go either way. A food processor: effort-free chopping! A food processor: a pain to clean! But anything that will make your life easier, on balance — such as an electric tin-opener, an onion slicer/dicer, a ring-pull can opener, a jar-lid gripper and so on — is worth it.

Use a slow-cooker or crockpot
A slow-cooker, as it's known in the UK, or crockpot, as it's called in the US, is a counter-top electrical pot that cooks food very slowly at a relatively low temperature. It's not a pressure cooker. You just chuck all the ingredients in — raw food and a liquid such as water, wine or stock — and leave it for hours unattended. People often start one cooking in the morning if they're going out and have a meal ready and waiting when they come home in the evening.

The fewer the ingredients, the easier the dishes are to prepare. Search on 'easy slow-cooker recipes', for example, and you'll find lots on the net. Phyllis Pellman's book, *Fix-It and Forget-It 5 Ingredient Favorites* is popular and gets good reviews, though it's American so presumably has US weights and measures.

Bear in mind that there'll be the smell of cooking food as long as it's on the go: possibly torture if you don't have a separate kitchen and tend to get peckish.

Try a double-sided grill

This product is an electric grill that sits on your counter and has a top and bottom plate that grills your food from both sides and so cooks twice as fast as a conventional grill. The grill plates are Teflon-coated and shaped to drain fat into a drip tray; they usually have a floating hinge so that the top plate will still lie flat on thicker items. You can get small grills suitable for one or two people. Importantly, they're said to be very easy to clean, and that's the feature that people say makes them less tiring to cook with.

Get lightweight crockery and pans

Do yourself a favour: forget that cast-iron skillet and get yourself some lightweight pans. Also consider buying lighter crockery. Test the weight in the store, if you can.

Use microwave steamer bags

These are sealable plastic bags with vents for steaming your vegetables in the microwave. Cooking with them takes just a few minutes and there's no washing up!

Use a perching stool

A perching stool is tall with non-slip feet so that you can perch on it, perhaps with it tipping forward, and have some support at the sink, hob or counter. However, perching stools can be hard work if you're having to brace your legs for balance. Also, if you have orthostatic intolerance, you're still basically vertical and such a stool might not help you much.

Use a microwaveable hot water bottle

OK, not so much a kitchen gadget as a gadget that you deal with in the kitchen, but microwaveable hot water bottles are great. Instead of heaving a heavy kettle about and trying to insert a torrent of boiling water into a small hole in a randomly shifting bag of rubber, you can just shove one of these in the microwave.

There are various types. I use the ones filled with wheat or millet, which adapt to your shape like a beanbag. I find they lose their heat quickly unless you insulate the side in contact with the air, so if you're not under a quilt with one, lay a folded jumper or towel or something on top of it to keep the heat in. Also, be sure to follow the instructions and when they're new, reheat them from cold several times to drive out the damp that they seem to hold at first.

If thermal-pack hot water bottles are heated in small microwaves and can't rotate freely, localised heating can melt the plastic. So check the sizes before you buy and when you heat the pack, make sure it's sitting well within the edges of the microwave plate.

Washing up

Use disposable plates and cutlery

Forget about being eco-friendly — if you're ill, you're ill, and disposable plates and/or cutlery can save you a lot of work if you're too sick to deal with washing up. Supermarkets sell small-quantity packs which are expensive so it's better to look on Ebay to buy in bulk from catering supply firms.

Even if you don't normally need disposables, it's good to have a stock of them in case you have a sudden bad patch and can't wash up.

Re-use cups and plates
If a plate has only had dry crumbs on it, sweep them off and use it for your next meal. Rinse your coffee cup and use it again. Obviously there's a limit but you can cut down on the whole washing-up rigmarole with this.

Line roasting and grilling pans
Line roasting tins or grilling pans with tinfoil (double-line them if necessary) so that you don't have to wash them. Another option is to use a Teflon liner sheet, which you can wash in the sink much more easily than you could a pan.

Line chopping-boards with kitchen towel
I keep one chopping-board for relatively dry vegetables such as mushrooms and carrots and protect it with a sheet of kitchen paper to keep it clean when chopping. At most, a bit of moisture might seep through but because the board will be protected on its next use by more kitchen towel, I wash it only very occasionally. Of course, the vegetables are always being chopped on the clean surface of a fresh paper towel.

Use freezer-to-microwave dishes
Freezer-to-microwave dishes are plastic, lidded containers that are freezer-safe and microwave-safe so you can heat

them straight from the freezer. I'm not mad on this idea because I'd be worried about chemicals leaching from the plastic into the food when the food is heated in the microwave: this is known to happen but it's hard to know whether it's to an extent that's harmful to health, in my opinion. I play safe and avoid them, but they're worth knowing about as an option.

Use non-stick cookware
Because life's too short.

Get a dishwasher
I'd marry my dishwasher if I could. Standing at the sink is very tiring if you have orthostatic intolerance; a dishwasher solves that problem. You can get compact dishwashers that sit on your kitchen top as well as slimline ones, so they're a possibility even in a small kitchen.

Soak your dishes before washing
Soaking your dishes before washing them can save a lot of brute force, especially with pans.

Let dishes air-dry
Put that tea-towel down! Fill a washing-up bowl with clean water and place it between the sink and the dishrack. Dip each item in it after you've washed it to rinse off the detergent.

5. HOUSEWORK

General cleaning

Keep things together that are used together
Store cleaning materials together in a bucket, bathroom cleaning stuff in the bathroom, and so on.

Give the bathroom sink a quick wipe
Keep paper towels in the bathroom and give the basin a quick wipe every now and then. It means you don't have to give it a full clean so often.

Wipe the bath while you're still in it
It's easier to stay in the bath until it has drained and then wipe it while you're still in it than it is to get out and bend over to scrub the waterline once it's all started to dry on. I don't have baths at all, partly to avoid ever having to clean the tub.

Use spray-and-rinse cleaning products
Hooray for these!

Leave cleaning products on long enough to do the work
Let chemistry take the strain: squirt the cleaner onto your sink and leave it to do its thing for a few minutes. You won't have to scrub so hard.

Use a bath mop to clean the bath

I didn't know that bath mops existed. They have long handles to save you bending. Search on Amazon or Ebay for 'bath mop' to find them.

Use wet wipes for cleaning and dusting

Wet wipes or baby wipes are powerfully cleansing. I cleaned most of a nasty black stain, possibly soot, from my nylon carpet using these. Who knows what they're doing to babies' bottoms but people use them to remove stains from sofas, hardened food from plates, scale from taps, the ring of grime from the bath, anything spilled on the floor, you name it.

They're also good for dusting because the dampness prevents the dust from spreading. Keep some in each room so you can grab one and deal with things as the need arises.

Use microfibre dusters

I think I did some dusting once. Tony Blair was still prime minister. So, not my area of expertise but I read about microfibre dusters a while back and got some for my home help to use. I had a little go with one and the texture was very peculiar: I felt as though it was trying to crawl up my hand. Although there are horror films that start like that (albeit not featuring dusters), there's no denying that microfibre cloths suck up the dust. You can slightly dampen them, which can help, and they're also excellent for buffing mirrors.

Keep turning the microfibre duster to use a clean area and don't use chemicals or cleaners with them.

Line the bathroom bin
Using small binliners for your bathroom pedal-bin keeps it nicer and makes it much easier to empty.

Keep dry waste out of the kitchen bin
You can empty your kitchen bin less often if you reserve it for food waste, which can be a huge help if it's not a task that you're always up to or if it's a long trip to the refuse-collection point. Put dry waste in another bin. Also, if you finish, say, a carton of soup, you can keep it on the counter until you've filled it up with food waste; this helps keep the rubbish compact so that your bin fills less quickly.

Floors

Hoover less often
I haven't been able to use a vacuum-cleaner for some years now and before I got a home help I just ignored the floor as the dust formed drifts against the skirting boards. Delightful! But it didn't seem to hurt me. So unless you have allergies that might be made worse by dust or have a carpet-moth problem, reconsider how often you really need to hoover.

Get a robot vacuum-cleaner
Because of the dust-dune issue, I got an iRobot vacuum-cleaner after a friend with laminate floors raved about hers. I had it for a couple of years and thought it did a great job on my carpets. My rug got so much cleaner that it

seemed to change colour. Take a look on YouTube. Not only can you see the iRobot adverts but you can see footage of people's kittens riding around on them. My vacuum-cleaner, the size of a dinner plate and about four inches tall, would amble randomly around my flat, gently nudging table legs with its rubber bumpers, and heading for its recharging station when it got tired. Its onboard computer knew where it had been and made sure that it covered everything, and it sang one merry little tune when it needed its dust container changing and another when it had finished the job.

In the end I sold it because I found it tiring to have to keep getting down to floor level to empty the dust receptacle, which was rather small, and because I'd decided to get a home help who could use an upright hoover. But if I was still on my own with the housework, I'd still have it.

There are several different robot vacuum-cleaners on the market now and they all look fairly similar, though prices vary enormously. Check out the reviews before you buy.

Get a robot floor-washer

A robot floor-washer is not something I've tried myself. They're similar to the robot vacuum-cleaners except that they mop your floors.

Get a lightweight hoover

If you put 'lightweight hoover' into Amazon's search engine, quite a few come up. Reading the reviews, it seems clear that some are light at the expense of power, so pay attention to reviews for any particular model that you're considering, especially any critical ones.

Get a Swiffer

The Swiffer seems to be one of those products that's huge in the US but completely unknown elsewhere. Jonah Lehrer's book *Imagine*, on the psychology of creativity, gives a highly dramatic account of the Swiffer's invention (well, maybe you had to be there). It's a floormop-cum-sweeper that has a handle assembly with a disposable cloth on the end: a dry, microfibre one, which picks up dust and dirt electrostatically, or a wet one pre-soaked with liquid cleaner, which mops. The latter saves you the whole thing of carting heavy buckets of water about and all the aggro of squeezing the mop out afterwards — you just throw the cloth away.

Swiffer provide refills of both kinds of cloth but many people save money by washing and re-using the dry cloths and using cheap wet-wipes to replace the proprietary wet cloths.

I told my home help the thrilling tale of the invention of the Swiffer and of its many glories and she bought one for herself, which she loves. Now I've got one for her to use on my floors and it does a good job.

The Swiffer people also do other products such as a wet-jet cleaner and a disposable duster on a stick so be careful that you're actually buying the sweeper starter kit with the wet and dry cloths. There are other, cheaper makes, including other brands of the cloth refills, all of which pop up on Amazon when you search on 'Swiffer'. They might also be worth a look.

Clean the kitchen floor with your feet
...but not just your feet. Soak a towel in hot water, wring it out and then drag it around the kitchen floor with your foot. Throw the towel in the washing machine when you've finished. Hang onto something stable while you're doing it, though.

Dust floors with your slippers
Mop slippers have a reusable microfibre cloth velcroed to the sole with lots of fluffy fingers that pick up the dirt from your hard floors as you walk about. Presumably you have to take them off every time you encounter a carpet. They freak me out because they look a bit centipede-ish. Don't let me stop you, though.

Laundry

Choose machine-washable clothes
It's best to avoid buying any clothes that need hand-washing or dry-cleaning.

Choose clothes the same colour
If most of your clothes are essentially beige, don't buy just the one bright green top because you'll be forced to handwash it to avoid the colour running into the rest of your laundry.

Use dye-catching products in the washing machine
Dylon's Colour Catcher and Vanish Oxi Action 2-in-1 Magnets are examples of chemical-impregnated sheets that you put in your machine wash to capture dye from strongly

coloured clothes that would otherwise stain your other items. I imagine they have their limits but I've heard good reports from friends who've tried them. Better than you standing at the sink handwashing your bright red jimjams because you've got nothing else to put them in the machine with.

Wear a t-shirt under hard-to-clean clothes
Some things take more effort to wash and iron (if iron you must), particularly sweaters and shirts. Wear a thin cotton t-shirt under these hard-work items so it's the t-shirt that needs washing often, not the other stuff.

Deodorise clothes in the sun
Turn not-quite-dirty but slightly sweaty clothes inside out and deodorise them in strong sunlight. I expect this tip came from someone in Arizona. If you live in Grimsby, I think you can pretty much forget about it.

Avoid scrubbing
It's easier to spray stain remover onto a stain, leave it to work for a while and then chuck the garment in the washing machine than wear your arm out scrubbing.

Bring the clothes airer to the washing machine
It may be easier to load things straight from the machine to the clothes airer. Or it may not. This works well for me if I have a lot of items because I have a lightweight A-frame clothes airer that doesn't collapse if I then pick the whole thing up and move it to a good drying spot. Just depends.

Lower the clothesline, raise the basket
If you use a clothesline, lower it while you're hanging up the washing and place the laundry basket on a chair to avoid stooping.

Ironing

Buy clothes that don't need ironing
Almost all my tops are jersey t-shirts or knitted sweaters. I've never ironed any of them. I put them on and the creases drop out. That's their job.

Surprisingly, creases also drop out of my jeans when they've been washed, so I never bother ironing them either. Experiment: you too may be emitting a magical ironing-field.

Hang clothes up
Even if they go in ironed, clothes can get creased in drawers, so hang everything up that you can, as long as it doesn't become a self-defeating crush.

Use the crease reduction/permanent press options on your washer or dryer
These seem to have been invented when I wasn't looking but apparently even people who have these options on their washers and/or dryers don't notice them. If you use them, don't overfill your machine because that causes wrinkles. As soon as the cycle ends, remove the clothes and

hang them up or fold them to prevent creases from developing.

Put a damp cloth in the dryer
I don't possess a washer-dryer so I can't vouch for this one, but it is alleged on the internet that if you stop the dryer early or place a wrinkled item in the dryer for five minutes with a damp cloth, your clothing will be ready to wear. Sounds plausible. Who knows?

Iron things by sitting on them
Perhaps the magical ironing-field that I mentioned earlier could be your bottom. Years ago, I read a memoir about trainee nurses in the 1950s who did the ironing by laying their slightly damp clothes flat on a table and sitting on them while drinking cups of tea and gossiping about men. I can't testify to the effectiveness of this one, as I haven't tried it. It all sounded very jolly, though.

Use a lightweight iron
Ironing? Why are you actually ironing? But if you must, try a lightweight iron.

Sit down while ironing
You should be able to adjust your ironing board low enough for you to sit on a chair while you iron.

Iron things while they're damp
Linen and cotton especially are hard to iron once they're dry. Iron them while they're still slightly damp. If they've already dried, moisten them by using the spray button on

your iron if there is one, or spray them with water from a plant-spray bottle.

Iron only what shows
If you're going to be wearing a sweater, only iron the collar and cuffs of your shirt; if you only wear trousers with a tunic, only iron the lower parts of the legs; if you're wearing a jacket, only iron the front of your shirt.

Changing bedlinen

Get a duvet
That's it. Just get a duvet. However, whereas the duvet is a brilliant invention, what were they thinking about with the duvet cover? Which brings me onto the following...

Use a topsheet under the duvet
Don't bother changing the duvet cover! Sleep between two sheets, with the duvet on top in a clean cover. When the bedding needs changing, just change the sheets: it's much easier. Eventually, the duvet cover will get dusty, like any surface in the home. You can shake the dust off, hoover it off with the brush extension on your vacuum-cleaner, or eventually wash the cover. But this method means that you can sleep in clean bedding without having to tackle the cover too often.

Don't lift the duvet high to change the cover
If you have orthostatic intolerance, keep your arms below your heart while doing this task by laying the cover on the bed and then inserting the duvet.

Get an easy-change duvet cover
Some duvet covers open on three sides rather than just the usual one. The whole cover hinges open, you lay the duvet flat on it, and do up the three sides using buttons or a zip. Easy! But they seem to be too specialised to be stocked in shops.

Googling has found me such covers by three companies selling direct online in the UK; Qande Duvet Covers, The Easylay Duvet Cover Company and All Zipped Up. I recommend caution in dealing with unfamiliar online enterprises. All Zipped Up, however, has one of its designs each with Amazon and House of Bath, who are, of course, well-known; they are also mentioned on a number of disability advice sites.

Outside the UK, searching on 'easy change duvet covers' should get you some results for your own country.

Another option would be for you or someone else with the skill and a sewing machine to adapt an existing cover.

Change the sheets less often
Remember at the beginning where I said, 'lower your standards'? Well, now's the time. I read on one online forum that people at an ME support group had a competition to see how long they'd managed to go without changing their sheets and the winner had managed six

months. However long you leave it, other people are leaving it longer, so don't feel bad!

Do change the pillowcases, though: they absorb oil from your hair and just changing them will help the whole bed experience seem much fresher.

Wear pyjamas and socks in bed

Wearing pyjamas and clean socks in bed will protect the sheets and help put off that evil laundry day.

Use a sleeping-bag liner

A sleeping-bag liner is basically a sleeping-bag made out of a sheet. If you sleep in one, you can just yank it out and shove it in the washing machine without needing to remake the bed, which is a major part of the trouble with sheets. If you find ready-made sleeping-bag liners too small, you can make your own (or get your own made) by folding a flat sheet in half and sewing together two of the sides.

6. OTHER ACTIVITIES IN THE HOME

Shopping from home

Online grocery shopping

This is the greatest advance that civilisation has made this millennium! What a fantastic thing.

In the UK, Tesco, Sainsbury's, Asda and Waitrose (via Ocado) deliver their groceries to your door (to your kitchen, if you want). After you've checked that the company delivers to your postcode, you register on their site, book a delivery slot to suit you, select your items, and that's it. A weekly shop that took me 40 minutes and a car journey when I was well now takes me 10 minutes online.

Time-slots for delivery are one hour for Sainsbury's and Waitrose, and two hours for Tesco and Asda so you don't have to wait in all day for your shopping. There's currently a minimum order of £25 for Asda and Sainsbury's and a £40 minimum order for Tesco and Waitrose. The delivery charge varies by company, time of day and size of order and ranges from zero to about £7; the average is probably about £3 or so, which means that someone delivers an entire week's shopping to your door for a bit more than the cost of a posh coffee.

Some of the supermarkets deliver more than just groceries with their 'grocery' service. They all offer computer printing paper, for example, which would be a ton weight to carry home yourself. It's well worth checking what else they have that you want.

Some companies don't offer delivery above the first floor as standard and even those that do can sometimes have drivers or local depots that are confused about their policy. If you live in a flat, call the company, tell them that you are disabled and need the driver to carry your shopping to your door, and check that they will do this. They should put a note on your account. If a driver ever turns up and doesn't seem to expect to deliver to you in this way, get back on the phone to sort it out. I've had to work through such confusion in the early days of my deliveries with some companies but it's easily been worth it: this delivery service alone has enabled me to remain independent in my own home.

Ebay and Amazon

Although there are plenty of online stores, Ebay and Amazon hold a gigantic range of items from a huge number of businesses, all of them striving to keep up their online reputations by getting positive reviews from customers. This gives me more confidence in ordering through them than through some company I've never heard of.

Also, unlike buying online direct from a load of sellers who would require you to register with them individually, you just register once with Ebay and/or Amazon and that's all your registration done. To buy, you just whack in your search terms, choose your item, hit the button and a few days later it gets delivered to your door. Very effort-saving.

Another advantage with Ebay is that it offers many cheap, tiny purchases that would elsewhere incur disproportionate delivery fees. For example, a £1.29 eyebrow pencil has free delivery on Ebay; delivery of any item under £40 from Boots costs £2.95. Because there's no big cost barrier with Ebay, using it for small items means you're not forced to wear yourself out with a trip to the shops.

If you're buying from Amazon, remember that many ME charities have an Amazon Affiliate button on their websites. Click through to Amazon from that button and the charity gets 5-9% of your spend during that session, at no cost to you.

Get chainstores to deliver

Is it a struggle to go to M&S for your socks? Then don't! Order online and get them delivered. Most big stores offer free delivery above a certain order value as well as free returns. Even if there is a delivery or returns charge, it's often small compared to what you might have spent on either transport (don't forget petrol costs and parking charges) or personal effort.

A further advantage is that if you try that pullover on in the store, you might not realise its full horror until you've got it home and seen it in natural light, by which time you've got to make another trip to return it and stand in a massive queue in the returns department. If it's been mailed to you, you can just mail it back.

Get your prescriptions delivered

Many local pharmacists will pick up your prescriptions from your GP's surgery and deliver them to your home for free. Outstanding! Stay at home and avoid getting coughed on.

Order library books online

OK, not so much shopping as borrowing, but anyway, this tip will save you a trip into town. Most library systems these days let you search your whole region's catalogue online at home and order books that will be delivered to your local library, for the same small reservation fee that you'd pay in the bricks-and-mortar library. Your library emails you when your books arrive.

Get library books delivered

Some libraries have volunteers who will deliver books, audiobooks, CDs and so on to your home. Some have a minibus to bring you to the library. A postcode lottery, my friends. Take a look at your library's website or give them a call to find out what's on offer.

Make your own Post Office

Ah, Christmas! Standing in an infinite queue to mail your parcels while the other customers sneeze their winter germs on you. No! You can do better.

Search on Ebay for 'digital kitchen postal scales', and for a fiver you will find the means to weigh a normal-size, not-gigantic package (leave 'kitchen' out of your search terms if you want to weigh enormous things). Download price information by googling on 'Royal Mail postage rates leaflet'.

You can buy postage online on the Post Office website but I prefer to buy a huge stock of stamps — say, twenty £1 stamps, fifty 10p stamps — from my local bureau a few times a year and just stick them on, not bothering about the odd penny here and there.

Keep stocked up
Make sure you've got plenty of basic necessities such as loo roll, toothpaste, washing-up liquid and so on in the house so that you never need to make an emergency trip for supplies when you might not be up to it. Keep a list somewhere prominent that you can add to when you notice you're running low on something so you don't get caught out.

Walking and carrying

Keep together what you use together
Save yourself a lot of wandering about and keep things that you use together in the same place: possibly in a container that you can carry to where you're going to do the activity. Buy duplicate items if that would help. For example, if you have one box for your stationery and another for your sewing kit, keep scissors in both.

Keep multiples of useful items in different rooms

Do you ever go into another room for a tissue? A pair of scissors? Whatever it is, buy several of it and keep one in every room where it's needed.

Use a bigger glass

Constantly going to and from the kitchen for a glass of water? Bigger glass!

Keep drinking water where you need it

If you're stuck in bed and the kitchen is some distance away, keep a large bottle or jug of water by your side so you don't have to make a special trip every time you need a drink.

Make up batches of tablets

Rather than take your bottles of supplements and pills out of the cupboard each time you need them, fill up a compartmentalised pillbox with several days' worth. You can get containers marked with the days of the week and with sections for morning, afternoon and evening.

Use a trolley to move things between rooms

Urgh, trolleys. Horrible wobbly things. But if you must, they can be handy for moving things from room to room. I suppose.

Have a chair or stool in every room

Wherever there's an activity that you normally do standing but could do sitting — for example, folding laundry straight out of the dryer in the utility room, cleaning your teeth in the bathroom — have a chair or stool there.

Take things from room to room when you're going anyway

Avoid special trips to transport things. If you're in bed and want to go to the kitchen to get a cup of tea, take your finished library book to the hall table on the way.

Declutter

Lots of jobs are easier if you have less stuff: dusting, finding things in cupboards, getting from one side of the room to the other, even just keeping your head straight. So if you don't need it, get rid of it.

Aim for one-floor living

If you find stairs seriously tiring, then pick the floor where you most need to be (possibly determined by the location of the bathroom or kitchen) and try to have what you need on that floor. You might even want to move your bed there.

Keep duplicate tools and supplies on both floors

If there are some jobs you do both upstairs and downstairs, keep more than one set of supplies on both floors: scissors, mops, brooms, buckets, dustpans, cleaning products, binbags and so on.

It might even be worth investing in a second (cheaper) hoover to avoid dragging one upstairs.

Throw laundry down the stairs

If your washing machine is downstairs, throw dirty linen down in pillowcases, rather than making extra trips.

I like this tip so much I wish I had some stairs to throw things down.

Get a stairlift
Getting a stairlift might be worth considering if you find your stairs a nightmare.

Visitors

Be upfront about your limits
If you invite someone to your home, tell them that you hope they'll understand that you can't last very long. Tell them how long a visit you can cope with. That way, they won't resent having made a two-hour round trip to spend twenty minutes with you when they could have seen you on their way to somewhere else another day.

Position a clock behind your visitor
A strategically-placed clock somewhere behind your visitor will save you constantly looking impolitely at your watch to check for the time when you'll have reached your energy limit.

Position a clock in front of your visitor
If it's a caller you can trust to understand your limits, they won't want to tire you out but, like you, they wont want to seem rude by checking their watch. A clock that they can easily see will solve the problem.

Get someone else to bring the visit to a close
Of course, all this ejecting of visitors can be done more gracefully if someone lives with you who can come in at a

pre-arranged time and remind you that it's time for you to stop before you get worn out.

Set a timer
All this tactful stuff about strategically-placed clocks and gentle reminders! Sometimes I think it would be better to have my massive oven timer go off after an hour so my visitor and I could have a good laugh about it, followed by an efficient departure.

Or maybe not. Time will tell...

Go out so you can leave when you want
One solution to the problem of visitors is not to have any. If you can meet friends at their place or at a cafe, you can simply leave when you need to.

Using the phone

Use the speaker facility while on hold
I would like to say that a lot of people don't realise that their phone has a speaker facility but maybe that was just me. But now I've found it, it's great! I no longer wear my arm out holding the receiver while stuck in a call queue. You make your call and if you're placed on hold you press the speaker button, hold it down, place the handset on the cradle and release the button to hear the other side through the speaker.

Use a hands-free headset
You can get a hands-free headset even for a landline phone if it has a headset port. Entering 'phone with headset' in Amazon's search box gives a few results.

Use a lightweight landline-handset
Some phones (I'm talking about you, 1970s retro phones) weigh a ton. Handset weight doesn't seem to be listed online in product details but it's something to be aware of when you're buying. If you have one delivered and it's too heavy, send it back.

Prepare a good excuse to get off the phone
If a phone call is going on a bit with someone who's difficult to shift and you're getting tired, you need a polite excuse ready to cut things short. I say I've heard the doorbell for my taxi, or that the timer has gone off and I've got to get something out of the oven.

Reading

Use a lap-desk or cushion to support your book
It's easier to rest your book on a cushion or a lap tray with a beanbag cushion rather than to hold it up yourself.

Use a bookholder to hold your book open
Hands-free! Bung 'book holder' into Amazon or Ebay and you'll find various types. I've used the Gimble and found it useful.

Get a book rest

There are a number of products, such as the Book Seat and the Peeramid, that let your book or e-reader recline like a spoiled prince upon an angled cushion with (unlike a spoiled prince) its pages pinned back so that you can read comfortably in bed. I suspect that both products might run into trouble with heavy or especially thick books.

Get a floor-standing book holder

You can get floor-standing holders for books and e-readers. They're not cheap! But if you do a lot of reading and want to have a good posture (something I waved goodbye to some time ago) while you're doing it, these can hold your book in a good position. Some can even hold your book upside-down so that you can read while lying down, though not everyone finds that the pages are well-held in that position.

Make a 'book bridge' for supine reading

For a few pounds you can get a transparent sheet of 4mm perspex cut to order on Ebay (search on 'perspex cut to size' or 'acrylic cut to size'). A 'plank' about 9" wide and a yard long can be propped up on supports, such as the backs of two chairs. You place your book or newspaper face down on the 'bridge' and lie beneath it to read. You have to reach up to turn the pages but that seems a small price to pay for a bit of entertainment during fully supine, head-flat rest.

Get an e-reader

There are pros and cons with e-readers. The big energy-saving benefit is that they're as light as a book but you don't have to hold any pages open. And if you want to carry more than one book with you, there's no extra weight with an e-reader.

Older-generation e-readers have pale grey screens and so offer less contrast between type and background than a conventional book or the newer readers such as the Kindle Paperwhite. You might want to try before you buy, or order from a supplier who offers quibble-free returns. Not being free to read where you can also lie down, or straining to read are going to drain your energy so you need to be sure your device suits you.

Use audiobooks

Audiobooks are great for when you're too tired to read, and skilled actors doing dramatic readings are often much better than your own voice droning on in your head.

Until recently, the white-hot cutting edge of audiobook technology was the audio-CD:
hugely expensive to buy, and scratched and weirdly sticky if you borrowed one from the library. Fortunately, things have moved on and audiobooks are now available as digital files. I highly recommend Audible, which is Amazon's new (to me, anyway) provider of audiobooks for download. A cheap subscription bags you an audiobook per month at paperback prices.

Let a Kindle read to you

The Kindle Keyboard and Kindle Touch currently have an 'experimental' text-to-speech feature that reads books aloud in a slightly Stephen Hawkingesque robot-voice, as you can hear on the demonstrations on YouTube. You can choose a male or female voice, speed it up or slow it down, and pause the reading.

It's not all roses. Read-aloud isn't available for all books. Some publishers disallow its use for certain titles, apparently to protect their audiobook sales, so it's worth looking into whether the kind of books for which you might want this feature allow its use. I find that many of the non-fiction and self-published books that I read are enabled for text-to-speech. The Kindle voice sometimes mispronounces things, inflects them oddly, and occasionally drives like a juggernaut over punctuation. However, the read-aloud facility allows you to continue to 'read' many books when you have to lie down and I find it useful.

If you're considering buying a Kindle for this feature, check whether it's still included. As an 'experimental' item, I wonder if it might be withdrawn at some point.

Household Emergencies

Prepare a list of emergency numbers
I only thought to create this section when I woke up one morning to find my kitchen flooded with water, and myself with adrenalin. People with ME don't recover from stress very quickly (I'm fine now, thanks) so help avoid panic induced exhaustion by having a list of emergency phone contacts. Include several numbers for tradesmen in case the first one you call isn't available — plumbers, electricians, gas engineers, locksmiths — as well as

numbers for your doctor, the local pharmacy, the hospital, NHS Direct, taxi companies, the local police, your home insurance emergency line and the gas-leak reporting service.

Start a logbook for your home

Even in a non-emergency, it can be tiring to try to track down a good tradesperson or dig out the details of a trusted one you've used before. I keep a logbook for my flat listing work that I've had done, who did it, the quality of the work, and whether they were pleasant, punctual and had bothered to mention that they were going to be three days late. Saves loads of energy in finding someone and also helps to avoid dealing with difficult people who might be exhausting.

7. OUT AND ABOUT

Shopping outside the home

Browse online beforehand
About to go into town to get nice new boots for the winter? So was I, until I looked online at what the shops in town were selling and decided it wasn't worth bothering. Big chainstores have all their stuff on their websites these days. If you can't afford a wasted trip, look online first.

Phone ahead to check your item is in stock
I still get caught out by forgetting to phone the store to check that the item I'm about to make a special trip to buy is in stock. Good job I'm writing this book. I'll highlight this one.

Order and collect
As the internet continues to wreak havoc on the high street, real-world shops are increasingly offering a click-and-collect service with which you place your order online and it's all gathered and packed ready for you to collect at the store. John Lewis, Marks and Spencer, Boots, the supermarkets, they're all at it. It's a free service and it saves you wearing yourself out in the store, but of course you've got transport costs, you've got to walk between your bus or

car and the store and back, and you've got to schlepp all your shopping back home, so consider whether home delivery would be better, if it's available. Still, worth knowing about.

Keep an emergency cash-stash
You don't want to have to go to the ATM if it's out of your way and you suddenly need some money. Keep some cash in the house.

Organise your shopping list by aisle
A shopping list that follows the order in which you'll encounter your items as you travel the aisles will save you a lot of pointless back-and-forth. Some of those supermarkets are huge.

Go shopping when it's quiet
Shopping in a crowd is harder work and standing in a checkout queue can be very tiring. If possible, make shopping trips when it will be quiet.

Use a backpack
Backpacks can be a lot less tiring for everyday shopping than using carrier bags, a handbag or shoulderbag.

Get a fabric or plastic handbag
...or manbag, I'm not judging. Much lighter than leather: they might not last as long, but better that they wear out than that you do.

Use a shopping trolley
Except for very small quantities of shopping, it's worth using a trolley, not just to put your shopping in but to lean on.

Ask an assistant to go upstairs for you
If you'd struggle to go upstairs for something you need in a store and there's no lift, ask an assistant if someone would fetch it down for you, or would at least phone up to check it's there before you make the effort. No need to get into the whole 'invisible illness' scenario. The line I use is, 'I have trouble with stairs'. No-one has ever argued with me.

Use store-provided wheelchairs or scooters
Some large stores and shopping malls provide wheelchairs or mobility scooters: contact them to check.

Put your basket down when queuing
I put my basket on the floor in a supermarket queue and as the line advances, I push the basket forward with my foot. No point in holding up a dead weight when you don't have to.

Appointments

Just say no
The problem with appointments is that the other person often isn't punctual. You turn up on time and you could be waiting ages. Or you may have to set off stupidly early on a bus to be sure of being on time yourself and end up having

to wait once you get there. Either way, just sitting can be exhausting.

So, see if you can do whatever it is via correspondence or the phone. For example, I can email my GP or leave a message for him to call me back at a convenient time if my problem doesn't require him to see me face to face. That saves me a two-hour nightmare of round-trip travel and the germ-ridden queue in the waiting room.

Ask for a home visit

Some NHS services are available as housecalls but it's patchy. Mobile NHS opticians will visit if you can't leave home without help and if you fulfil some other conditions, such as being at risk of glaucoma or having a low income: google on 'optician home visits'. Dentist home visits seem a patchier service but googling and a bit of phoning in your local area could pay off. Home physiotherapy may be available via a GP referral and if you need blood tests or a throat swab, your GP may be willing to send a phlebotomist or nurse to you. Don't be shy about asking for any of these services if you need them.

It's not just health services that might offer home visits. Hairdressers, mortgage advisors, accountants: whoever you need to see, it's worth asking if they'll come to your house if your business can't be conducted by phone.

Explain your situation in advance

If you can't avoid going to an appointment and you think you might be in for a long wait at the other end — hospitals! — and would find it difficult to cope, then phone the service in advance. Explain that you have problems sitting for long periods of time because of a health condition and that it would help you cope if you could sit in their waiting room with your feet up, or maybe lie down somewhere, or be seen as soon as you get in even if it's not your turn.

Be careful with the latter idea. Some people can be very rigid in their thinking and can react angrily to a suggestion that you want to 'jump the queue' before it has really sunk in with them that it's possible to be too ill to cope with a queue. I usually explain that I'm largely confined to bed and first present the list of awkward requests to have my feet up or to lie down while waiting so they can grasp the severity of the problem. If they can't accommodate me, I then say something like, 'Under normal circumstances I wouldn't ask this because I don't want to be jumping any queue but it's really so physically difficult for me to sit for long, that if you think it's appropriate, perhaps it would be possible to ask Mr/Ms/Dr X if they could see me as the next person/patient so that I can go home straight away and rest and get out of your way. I really don't want to shove in but...' and so on.

Ask to wait in a side-room at the doctor's office

Ironically, a doctor's waiting room can be one of the hardest places for someone with ME to be: a potentially long period of sitting plus exposure to other patients' infections that might hit you extra hard if you get them. If your doctor is sympathetic, discuss whether you could wait in an side-room until called, preferably one with an examination couch where you can lie down.

Ask for a wheelchair at the hospital
Hospitals are huge. You can walk for miles. Contact the hospital in advance and ask about a wheelchair.

Travel and mobility

Get a wheelchair or mobility scooter
Now would be a good time to remember what I said at the beginning about these adaptations not necessarily being forever! No-one can be thrilled at the realisation that they need a wheelchair but using one can help you get a better balance between rest and exertion that might help you to recover. I'll admit it's not exactly like getting your first pony, though.

Even if you just rent or borrow a wheelchair for a short period for a try-out or to visit a particular place, they can be a great help. You can get powered models and properly padded ones with pneumatic tyres that don't shake you to bits over rough ground. In the UK, the Red Cross loan them and you can ask your GP to prescribe you one.

Get a reclining wheelchair
I've seen reclining wheelchairs recommended for people with severe orthostatic intolerance who need to lie down frequently. Sounds like a plan.

Get a disabled parking badge
In the UK, at least, you don't even have to own a car to get a disabled parking badge: you can use yours in any car in

which you're travelling. A huge help. Apply to your local council.

Take a taxi

For those of us who are either hard-up or tightfisted, taking a taxi can seem unthinkable but sometimes it just makes sense.

Break up long journeys

You can take breaks during a long car journey by stopping occasionally and lying down in the back. An overnight hotel stay is also an option for especially long distances.

Lie down for long car journeys

If, as a passenger, you find it hard to sit for long in a car, your only option may be to travel lying down on the back seat on a folded duvet with a pillow or two for comfort.

In the UK, any occupant of a motor vehicle must wear a seatbelt if one is fitted, but if your health condition prevents you from wearing one, you can ask your doctor for a medical exemption certificate and must show it to the police if challenged. Car insurers may need to be informed if someone is travelling while not restrained. Seatbelts, of course, protect not only the passengers in the rear but also the people in the front whom they might hit if there's a crash, so it's a matter of weighing the pros and cons.

Travel light

If you're travelling to stay away from home, pack the absolute minimum so that you're not carting heavy bags about. Just travel with the basics, if you can: mini-sized toiletries, enough clean underwear to see you through, a few t-shirts.

Keep duplicate items at frequent destinations
If there's someone you often go via public transport to stay with, ask if you can leave a few things that you need for every visit, to lighten your luggage. When I could still travel by train I kept toiletries, pyjamas and underwear at my parents' house, and kept a list of those items at home so that I could remember what I didn't need to take with me.

Mail luggage to your destination
I twice moved flats by mailing boxes of my belongings to myself at my new home but on a smaller scale I used to post a box full of everyone's Christmas presents to my parents' home rather than struggle with bags on the train. You can mail your clothes and anything else you need. You might want to insure the package!

Take only cabin luggage when flying
If your journey is a bit more ambitious than a local bus-ride and you're flying, take only cabin luggage so that you don't have to wait at the carousel for it later. The less luggage, the easier the journey.

Order a wheelchair at the airport
There's a lot of standing about in lines at airports. Order a wheelchair for both ends of your journey.

Resting outdoors

Sit wherever you can in an emergency
If you run out of steam when you're outdoors and there's no public bench, sit on a wall or nip into a shop that has chairs, or, if you have to, sit on the kerb. This is why I never wear white trousers!

Carry a portable cushion or seat
You can buy an inflatable cushion to keep in your bag for when you need to rest, or a lightweight portable seat with a back, or a walking-stick seat, which unfolds to form a tripod with a seat on top. If you fancy being like a retired colonel on a grouse-shoot, you could get a shooting-stick — a walking-stick with a handle that unfolds to form a seat and a sharpened point at the other end that can be stuck firmly in the ground.

Take a lightweight rug to lie down on
If it's the summer and you're going somewhere such as a park, where there's a grassed area, take a lightweight rug so you can lie down for a rest if you need one. Roll up your coat or sweater to use as a pillow. People will just think you're sunbathing!

8. THREE LAST GENERAL STRATEGIES

Keep finding out about new products

I've been amazed, while writing this book, what products have been invented that make life easier for everyone, not just those of us with health problems. Microfibre hair towels! Long-handled bath mops! Astronaut shampoo! Text-to-speech software! Complete news to me.

Once we buy a product, we can be a bit too loyal and still be using it decades later, not noticing that something better has come out. So if a particular task is giving you problems and my suggestions here haven't helped, start researching on the internet. You might find a useful new invention.

Brainstorm!

Inevitably, there'll be something you want to do that I haven't suggested any tips for. So brainstorm! Get your friends to brainstorm! Google! Think like a Martian! There's got to be a better way to do it.

Use online resources

Some of the most useful sources for this book have been online ME forums such as Phoenix Rising (perhaps the largest, with a specific section for discussing lifestyle adaptations), Prohealth and ME/CFS Forums. You don't have to be alone wondering how to solve a particular practical problem caused by your illness: there are plenty of people on those sites who have faced the same issues and who will have helpful advice. You don't have to give your real name as your username so don't be shy about registering and posting a question.

9. REASONS TO BE CHEERFUL

There will, I hope, come a day when none of us will need to worry about any of this stuff. As I write, it's the most promising time for ME research that I've seen in my long years of illness. In 2009, the possibility that the retrovirus XMRV might be responsible for the disease brought world-famous, top-flight scientists to join the hunt for a cause. XMRV has now been ruled out but that research momentum has snowballed. Professor Ian Lipkin, the world's foremost virus-hunter, is conducting a study looking at gene expression and a wide range of pathogens in a large, well-defined sample of people with ME. The cancer drug Rituximab has appeared highly effective in many ME patients in a pilot study in Norway; a Norwegian confirmatory trial is already underway and others are planned in the US and the UK. New, high-tech research institutes and collaborative networks are springing up and the pace is gathering.

Suddenly the future is much brighter and the time seems closer when you and I won't need a book like this. I look forward to a mass bonfire of the paperback version.

Until then, I wish you good health!

Printed in Great Britain
by Amazon